FIT
BABY

8 EXERCISE ROUTINES
FOR BABY'S FIRST YEAR

DARCI AND TY WISE

ISBN: 978-0-692-71093-7

Printed in the United States of America

Book design by Jean Boles
jean.bolesbooks@gmail.com

For Levi and Landon

Contents

About the Authors...1

Introduction...2

General Guidelines...4

Helpful Tips 6

Part One: The Exercises 8

    Stretches 8

    Baby Grip...8

    Plank Position 8

Month One Exercises 10

    Tummy Time..10

    Bicycle Kicks...11

    Butterflies..12

    Pull-ups 13

    Forearm Planks 14

    Punches 15

    Chin to Floor Stretch...16

    Ear to Shoulder Stretch...17

    Leg Stretch 18

    Chin Lift Stretch 19

    Back Stretch 20

Month Two Exercises 21

    Inside-Out Kicks 21

Month Three Exercises 22

    Sit-ups 22

    Guided Sitting 23

Month Four Exercises 24

    Guided Standing 24

Month Five Exercises 25

    Crawling Position 25

    Planks 26

Month Six Exercises 27

    Toe to Nose Touch 27

Month Seven Exercises 28

    Guided Walking 28

Part Two: The Routines 29

Month One Workout 30

Month Two Workout 31

Month Three Workout 32

Month Four Workout 33

Month Five Workout 34

Month Six Workout 35

Month Seven Workout 36

Month Eight Workout 37

About the Authors

Darci and Ty Wise are both entrepreneurs and public school teachers in Western Pennsylvania. They have been married for five years and live with their two young children. They are expecting another child in September 2016. Darci and Ty are advocates of a strong family, and they love being parents above anything else.

Ty has been involved with fitness since age seven as a successful athlete and later as a varsity wrestling coach, from which he has currently taken a break to raise a family.

Introduction

*W*hen we had our first baby we were excited, overwhelmed, and petrified all at the same time! Although it was nothing to be alarmed about, we noticed that our newborn son was having trouble keeping his neck straight. When lying down in his crib or even in our arms, he would always tilt his head to the same side. We eventually realized that this was a result of being cramped in a certain position in the womb.

My husband saw this as a problem that could be solved, so when our son was about one month old, Ty decided to try some neck stretches with him. Ty did the stretches with the baby a few times a day, and within a week or so he realized that the stretches were helping! The baby began holding his neck straighter because the neck muscles on both sides had become stronger.

Now to be honest, the baby wasn't too crazy about the neck stretches, especially at first. So my husband added in some other moves to the stretching sessions for variety. Needless to say, the stretching sessions evolved into baby workouts. After doing some research and using his own background in sports and coaching, Ty made the routines more detailed and more organized. As the baby grew capable of more and more activity, the workouts also changed regularly.

We continued exercising our son until he was about eight months old. The routines and exercises were such an important part of our first-year journey with him. When we had our second son, we didn't think twice about pulling out the old routines and using them again. Both of our boys are strong, flexible, and very spatially aware.

We know from personal experience that the Fit Baby workout routines will be incredibly beneficial to the physical health of your child. But more importantly, we hope that this will be a special bonding opportunity for you and your baby!

Darci & Ty Wise

General Guidelines

❶ Start exercising your baby as soon as he/she turns one month old. The early months are especially important for developing flexibility and strengthening muscles.

❷ Work out your baby once a day, every day. It's a great way to spend time together!

❸ Be very gentle when exercising your baby, especially in the first two months.

❹ None of the exercises should be painful for your baby. Sometimes your baby may show resistance to a certain move, and that is completely normal. If you feel your baby is miserable, use your best judgment and decrease the number of repetitions for that particular exercise, or change to another exercise entirely.

❺ Some exercises are omitted from the routines as the baby surpasses the need for them. Ultimately, it's up to you whether or not you think your baby has surpassed a particular exercise. Simply skip that exercise and move on to the next one in the routine.

❻ Fit Baby exercise routines are only meant to be a tool. Feel free to shorten workouts, change the order, etc. to meet your baby's individual needs.

❼ Always remember that your baby's safety is the number one priority!

Helpful Tips

- ➤ Be patient. Not all babies will respond with complete and utter joy when doing some of the exercises, especially at first. The more you exercise your baby, the more your baby (and you!) will be comfortable with it.

- ➤ If your baby gets upset, return to the Bicycle Kicks for as long as necessary. Then, either proceed with the rest of the routine or end for the day.

- ➤ When doing any of the stretches, your baby should be able to complete the full stretch with little resistance. If there is a lot of resistance or difficulty, gently stretch the baby as far as he/she can go, and try to go a little further every couple of days.

- ➤ Sometimes babies can get very hungry after exercising. Be prepared for a nursing or bottle session after you're finished, especially if it's close to a mealtime.

- ➤ If you have other young children in the home, get them involved in the workouts, too! They can work out on their own at their own level, or they can help exercise the baby (with plenty of parental guidance, of course).

- ➤ In some of the routines you will see "Bumbo Time." Bumbo refers to a special baby seat that you can purchase at any major retailer. If you don't want to purchase the seat, you will need to guide your baby in a sitting position by keeping your hands behind their back and repositioning them as necessary.

➢ To make the workouts more fun for your baby (and for you), play some music in the background. Pandora is a great website you can access on your computer or mobile device that has free streaming radio, including baby and toddler stations.

Part One: The Exercises

It is very important that you understand all of the exercises and read the following before starting the routines. Each exercise includes a brief description and a detailed illustration showing how to perform the exercise. All of the exercises are meant to improve your baby's flexibility, strength, and balance.

Stretches

There are several different types of stretches used in the routines. The ear to shoulder and chin to floor stretches can be skipped unless your baby has a stiff neck from birth (known as torticollis). The other stretches (chin lift, leg stretch, back stretch, and toe to nose touch) are beneficial to all babies.

Baby Grip

In many of the exercises, you will find that there is a specific way to grip your baby's hands. When your baby is young, the grip is more closed to offer a lot of support. The stronger your baby becomes, the looser the grip will be (For example, rather than the baby gripping your entire hand, he/she may only need to hold on to one finger, and thus is doing most of the "work".)

Plank Position

After your baby graduates from the forearm plank, he/she will do more of a standard plank position by supporting themselves on their hands. Where you hold and support your baby changes as your baby becomes stronger. You will support your baby at the hips in month five, at the thighs in month six, and finally, at the knees in month seven.

Pull-ups

Beginning in month five, you will begin pulling your baby all the way up to a standing position rather than a sitting position. Try to let your baby do most of the work by using a looser grip (baby holding thumb only), particularly when your baby is coming up from a squat to a stand.

Month One Exercises

Tummy Time

Directions:

❶ Place baby on belly for a designated amount of time and reposition if necessary.

Note: Tummy Time is so important because young babies can develop plagiocephaly (also known as "flat head syndrome") from spending too much time on their backs. Setting aside time for babies to be on their bellies also encourages babies to lift their heads off the ground, which will strengthen their neck muscles.

Tummy Time is omitted in the routines after month five because babies are typically rolling over at least one way by then, and thus spending enough time on their tummies on their own.

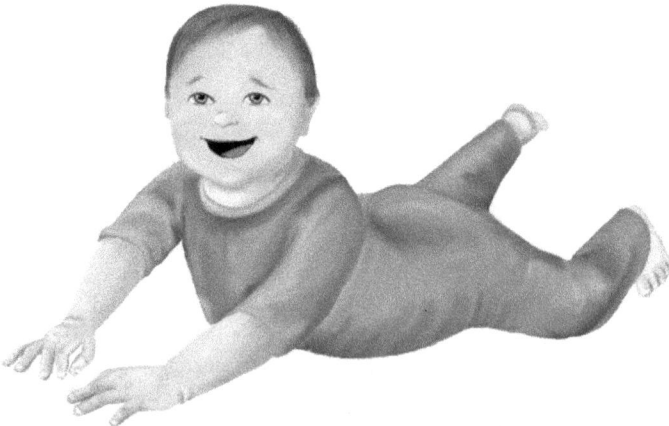

Month One Exercises

Bicycle Kicks

Directions:

❶ Place baby on back.

❷ Hold baby's ankles and push one leg toward baby's chest while gently pulling the other leg toward you.

❸ Alternate legs at a fast pace so that it looks like baby is riding a bicycle.

Note: As previously stated in Helpful Tips, anytime baby seems uncomfortable during the routines, return to the bicycle kicks for as long as desired. This is also a great exercise to help relieve any baby tummy pain (such as gas or constipation).

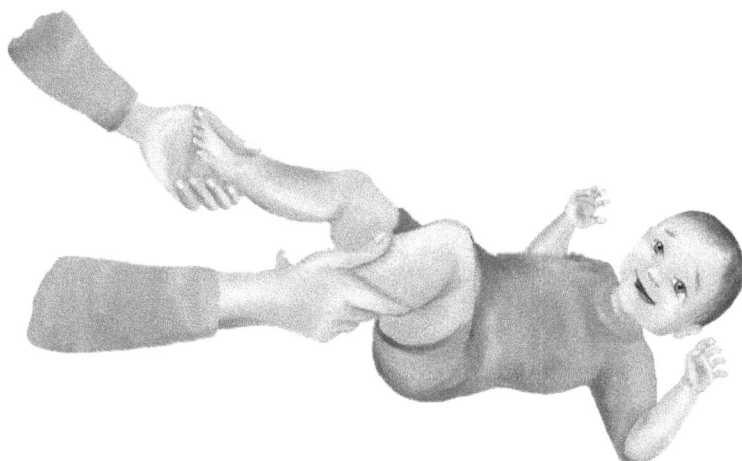

Month One Exercises

Butterflies

Directions:

❶ Place baby on back.

❷ Hold baby's wrists, with baby gripping your thumbs, and spread both arms out to sides.

❸ Bring baby's arms inward towards chest so that fists lightly touch, and spread arms out to sides again.

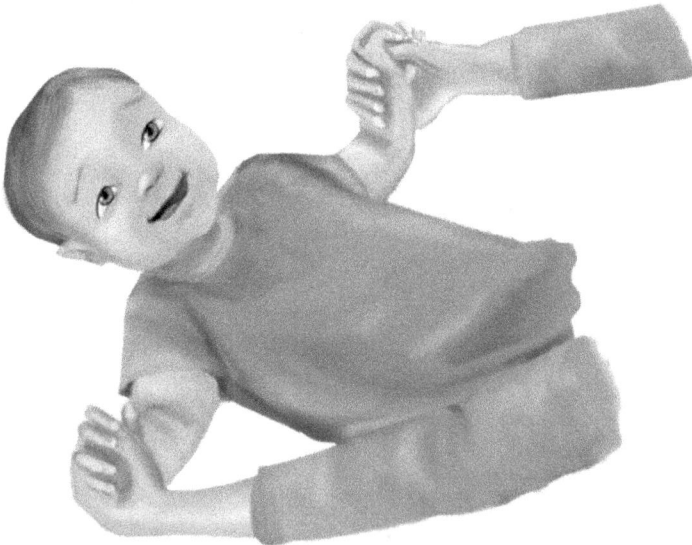

Month One Exercises

Pull-ups

Directions:

❶ Place baby on back.

❷ Hold baby's wrists, with baby gripping your thumbs, and slowly pull baby up to a seated position.

Note: Beginning in month five, baby is pulled up to a standing position rather than a sitting position.

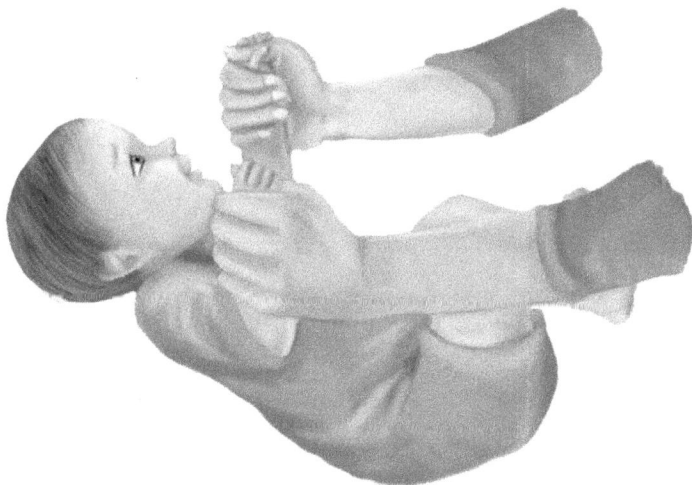

Month One Exercises

Forearm Planks

Directions:

❶ Place baby on belly.

❷ Place baby's elbows under shoulders so that forearms are flat on floor.

❸ Lift baby's hips slightly to form a 45-degree angle with floor and hold.

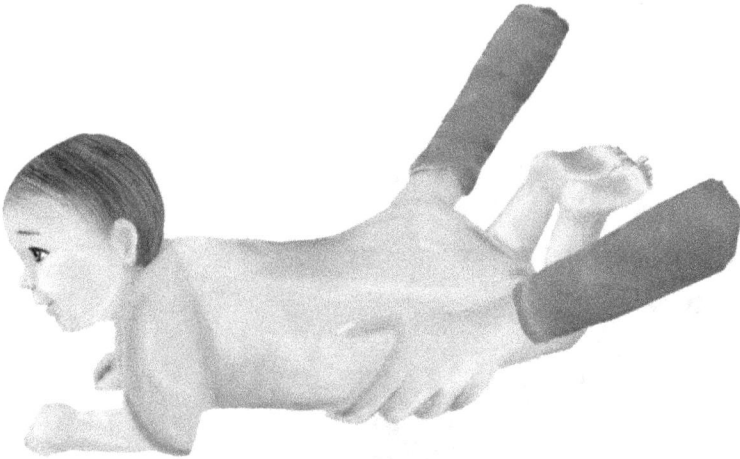

Month One Exercises

Punches

Directions:

❶ Place baby on back.

❷ Hold baby's wrists, with baby gripping your thumbs, and gently pull one arm toward you while pushing the opposite arm in to baby's shoulder.

❸ Alternate arms.

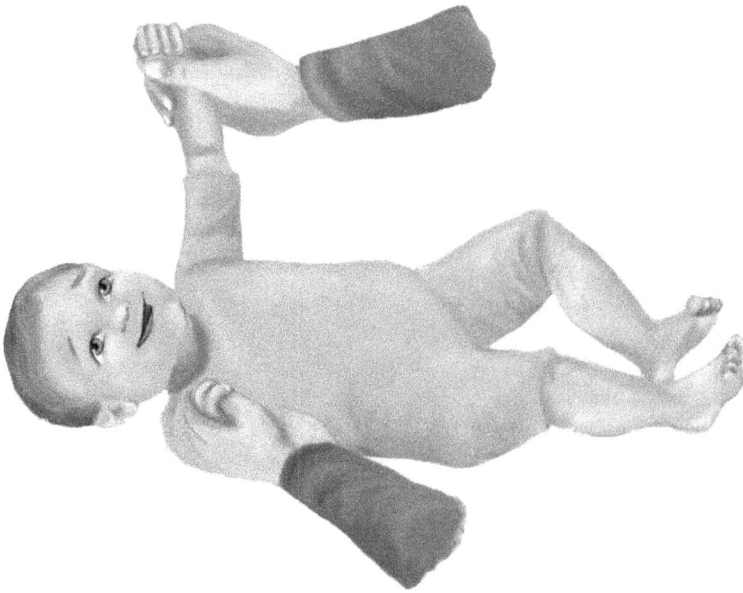

Month One Exercises

Chin to Floor Stretch

Directions:

❶ Place baby on back.

❷Turn baby's head to one side so that side of chin is slightly touching floor and hold.

❸ Repeat on opposite side.

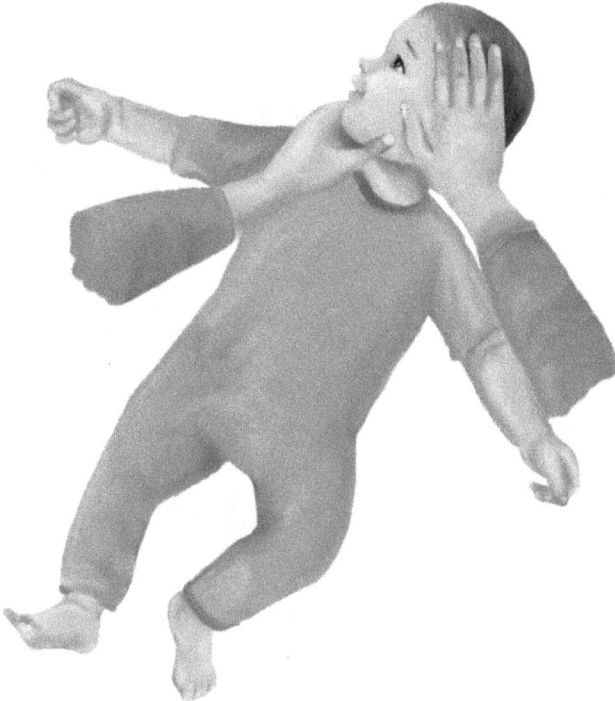

Month One Exercises

Ear to Shoulder Stretch

Directions:

❶ Place baby on back.

❷ Tilt baby's head so that ear is slightly touching shoulder and hold.

❸ Repeat on opposite side.

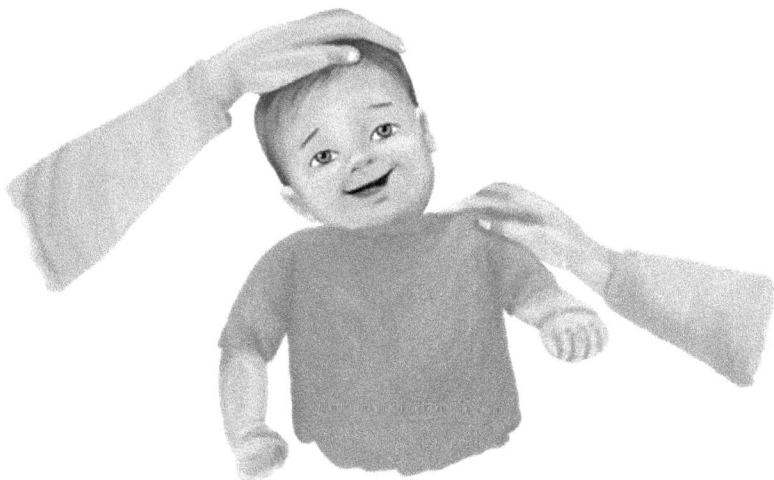

Month One Exercises

Leg Stretch

Directions:

❶ Place baby on back.

❷ Pull baby's legs toward you and gently press down at knees to straighten and hold.

Note: This is a great stretch for young babies because their legs are somewhat bent from being in the fetal position.

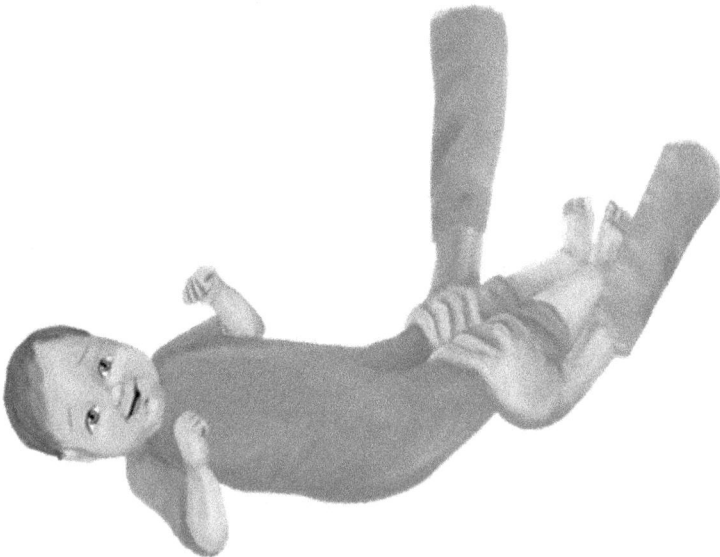

Month One Exercises

Chin Lift Stretch

Directions:

❶ Place baby on belly.

❷ Cup baby's chin and gently lift up so that baby is looking straight ahead and hold.

Note: When your baby has mastered lifting his/her head off the ground (90-degrees from the floor), there is no need to perform this stretch.

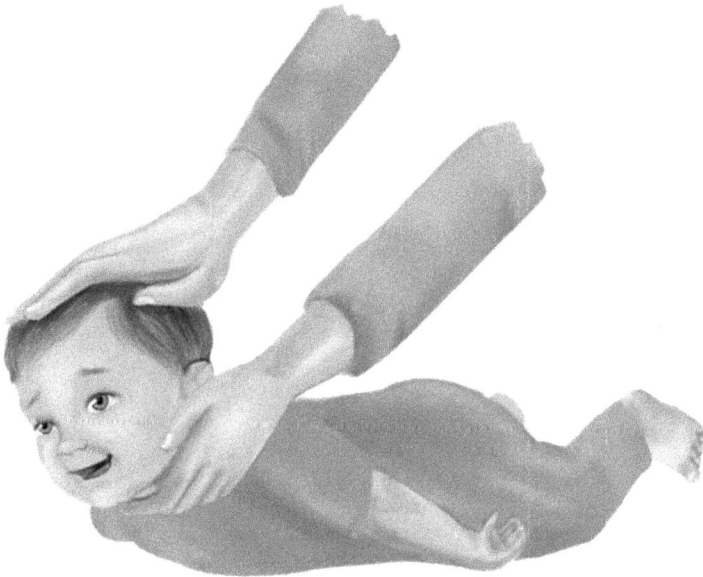

Month One Exercises

Back Stretch

Directions:

❶ Place baby on back.

❷ Place one hand under small of baby's back and gently push up.

❸ Let baby arch back naturally, just barely touching floor with head and hold.

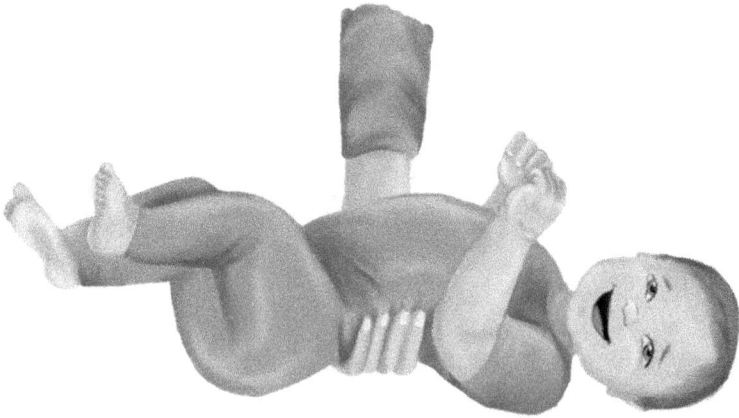

Month Two Exercises

Inside-Out Kicks

Directions:

❶ Place baby on back.

❷ Grip baby's feet and move one leg up toward baby's shoulder; bring it back down alongside body in a semi-circular motion to starting position.

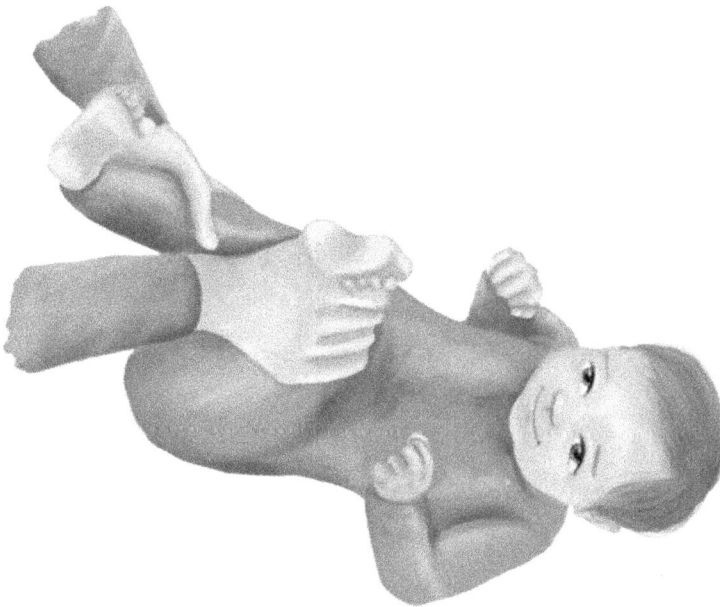

❸ Alternate legs.

Month Three Exercises

Sit-ups

Directions:

❶ Place baby on back.

❷ Hold baby's wrists, with baby gripping your thumbs.

❸ Pull up to a seated position and slowly bring back down onto back.

Note: This exercise is repeated in an up and down motion (looking like an adult sit-up) with a closed grip.

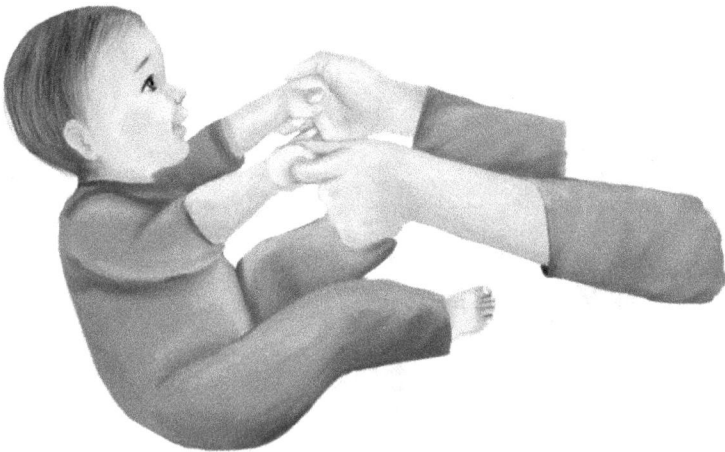

Month Three Exercises

Guided Sitting

Directions:

❶ Place baby in a seated position.

❷ Hold baby's wrists, with baby gripping your thumbs and balance. Reposition if necessary.

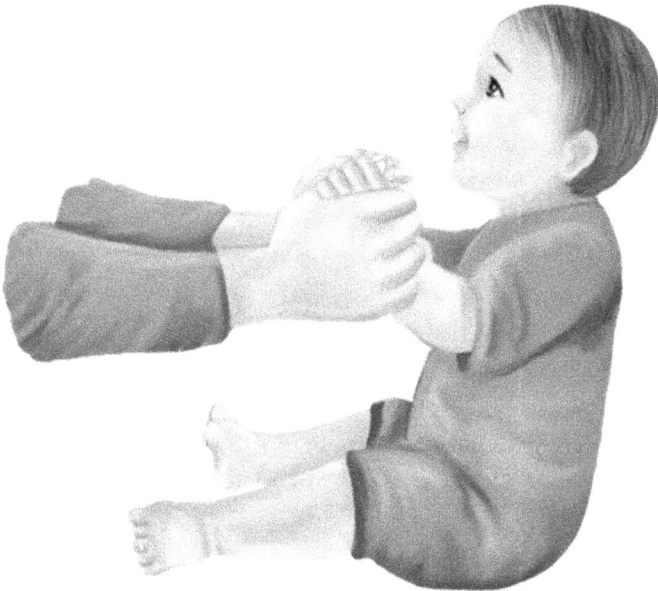

Month Four Exercises

Guided Standing

Directions:

❶ Pull baby up to a standing position.

❷ Hold baby's wrists, with baby gripping your index fingers and balance. Reposition if necessary.

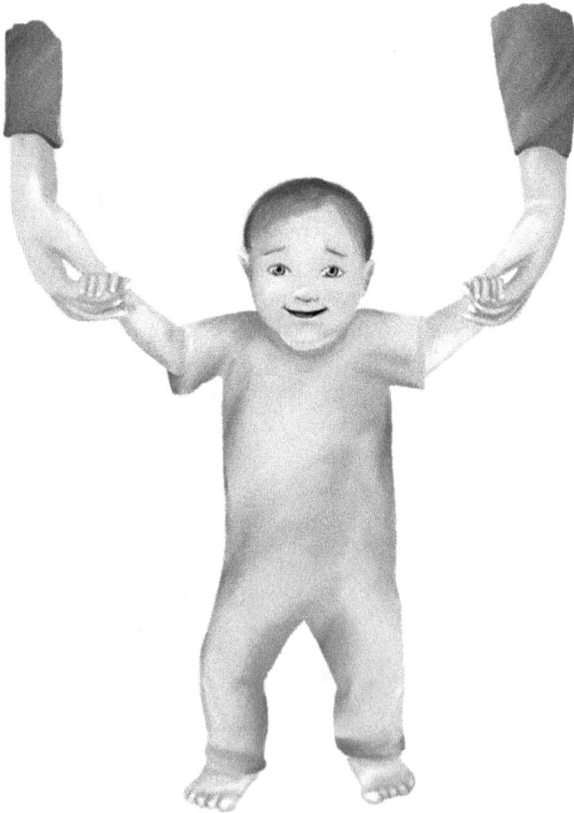

Month Five Exercises

Crawling Position

Directions:

❶ Place baby in a crawling position.

❷ Support baby at thighs and hold. Reposition if necessary.

Note: If your baby is already crawling, there is no need to perform this exercise.

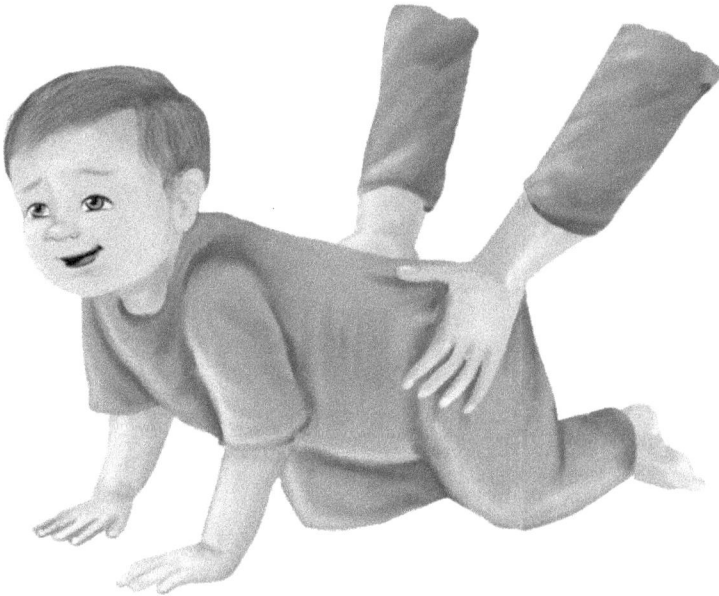

Month Five Exercises

Planks

Directions:

❶ Place baby on belly.

❷ Lift baby's hips and let baby support him/her self on hands with head facing forward and hold. Reposition if necessary.

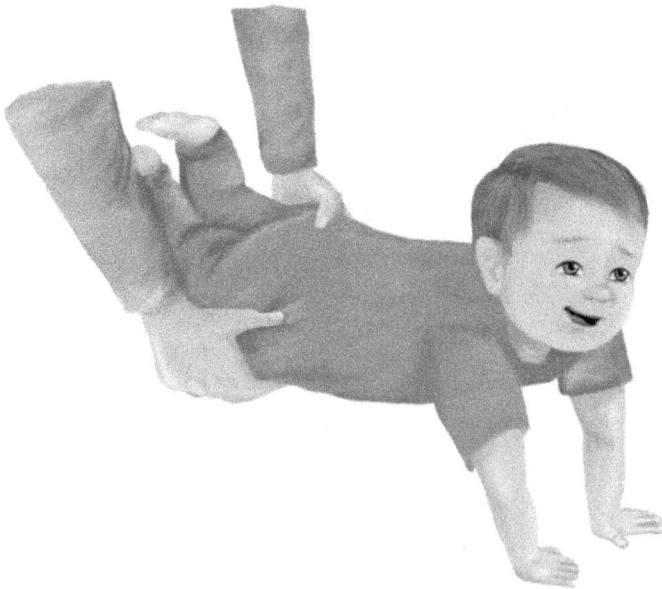

Month Six Exercises

Toe to Nose Touch

Directions:

❶ Place baby on back.

❷ Grip baby's feet, and with knees slightly bent, pull one leg up so baby's toe just barely touches nose.

❸ Repeat on opposite side.

Note: This is not a stretch that you hold for a certain amount of time; toe comes up to nose and then it is released.

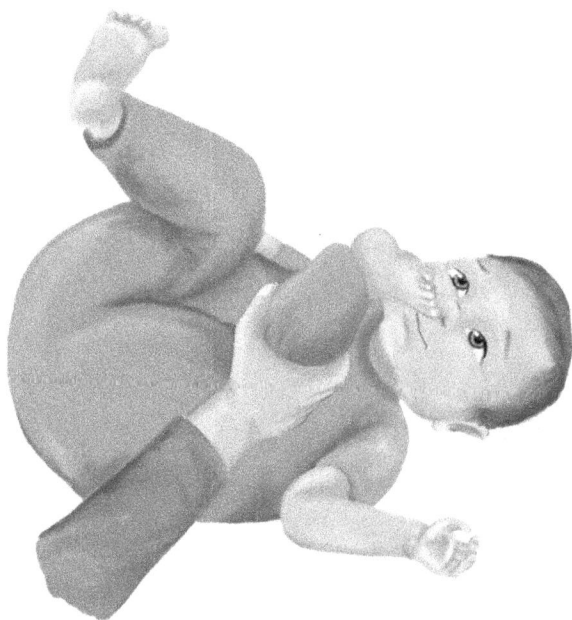

Month Seven Exercises

Guided Walking

Directions:

❶ Place baby in a standing position.

❷ Hold baby's wrists, with baby gripping your index fingers, and walk baby by pulling up gently on each arm and also moving forward slightly.

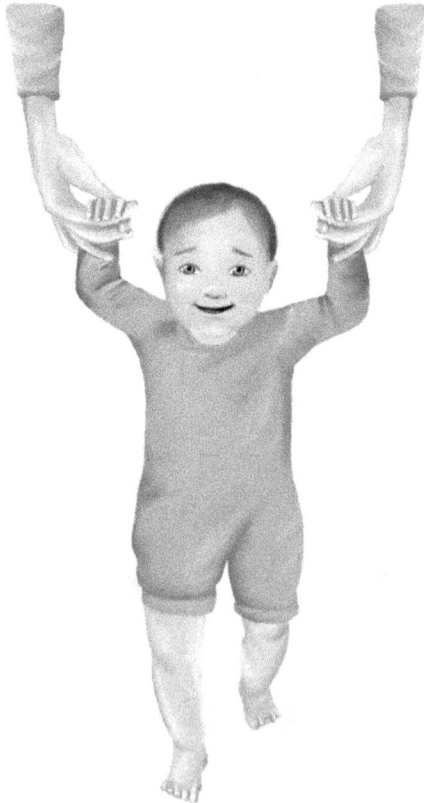

Note: Some babies may completely resist this exercise, and that is perfectly normal. If this happens, try guided walking again in the eighth month.

Part Two: The Routines

*T*here are a total of **8 Exercise Routines**. Baby can begin the routines at one month old and continue them until nine months. There are no additional routines after that because most babies are usually doing enough on their own at that point. You can always continue exercising your baby using the routines if you wish to do so!

In the routines, each exercise is listed with the number of repetitions (20xs) or the amount of time (20 sec) to do the exercise. This is just a guideline; you may decrease the number of repetitions or amount of time whenever you feel it necessary.

Also included in the routines are some of baby's first-year milestones. Physical milestones are already part of each routine, but additional ones are listed in case you want to add them to your session. The activities are based on what your baby *should be able to do* and *will probably be able to do* by the end of that particular month. Some milestones are repeated for more than one month because not all babies reach them at the same time. If your baby has mastered the milestones listed in the current month, feel free to begin working on the next month's milestones. If you're ever concerned about your baby's progress, speak with your pediatrician.

Month One Workout

1. Tummy Time 1 min
2. Punches 15xs
3. Butterflies 15xs
4. Bicycle Kicks 20 sec
5. Leg Stretch 5 sec
6. Punches 10xs
7. Butterflies 10xs
8. Bicycle Kicks 20 sec
9. Ear to Shoulder Stretch 5 sec
10. Pull-Up and Sit 1 min
11. Forearm Plank 10 sec
12. Bicycle Kicks 20 sec
13. Back Stretch 5 sec
14. Pull-Up and Sit 1 min
15. Chin Lift Stretch 5 sec
16. Bicycle Kicks 20 sec
17. Chin to Floor Stretch 5 sec

Estimated Time: 7 minutes

INCLUDED MILESTONE ACTIVITIES
On tummy, lift head briefly or lift head 45 degrees
(Tummy Time)

SUGGESTED MILESTONE ACTIVITIES
Follow an object in an arc six inches above face to midline

Month Two Workout

1. Tummy Time 2 min
2. Punches 20xs
3. Butterflies 20xs
4. Bicycle Kicks 20 sec
5. Leg Stretch 5 sec
6. Punches 10xs
7. Butterflies 10xs
8. Bicycle Kicks 20 sec
9. Ear to Shoulder Stretch 5 sec
10. Pull-up and Sit 1 min
11. Forearm Plank 10 sec
12. Inside-Out Kicks 10xs—*new exercise*
13. Back Stretch 5 sec
14. Pull-up and Sit 2 min
15. Forearm Plank 10 sec
16. Chin Lift Stretch 5 sec
17. Bicycle Kicks 20 sec
18. Chin to Floor Stretch 5 sec

Estimated Time: 9 minutes

INCLUDED MILESTONE ACTIVITIES
On tummy, lift head 45 degrees (Tummy Time)

ADDITIONAL MILESTONE ACTIVITIES
Follow an object in an arc six inches above face to midline
or past midline

Month Three Workout

1. Tummy Time 3 min
2. Punches 25xs
3. Butterflies 25xs
4. Bicycle Kicks 20 sec
5. Leg Stretch 5 sec
6. Punches 10xs
7. Butterflies 10xs
8. Bicycle Kicks 20 sec
9. Ear to Shoulder Stretch 5 sec
10. Pull-up and Sit 1 min
11. Forearm Plank 15 sec
12. Inside-Out Kicks 10xs
13. Back Stretch 5 sec
14. Sit-ups 3xs—*new exercise*
15. Forearm Plank 10 sec
16. Chin to Floor Stretch 5 sec
17. Bicycle Kicks 20 sec
18. Chin Lift Stretch 5 sec
19. Bumbo Time 3 min—*new exercise*

Estimated Time: 11 minutes

INCLUDED MILESTONE ACTIVITIES
On tummy, lift head 45 degrees or 90 degrees
(Tummy Time)

ADDITIONAL MILESTONE ACTIVITIES
Follow an object in an arc six inches above face past
midline or from one side to the other

Month Four Workout

1. Tummy Time 4 min
2. Punches 30xs
3. Butterflies 30xs
4. Bicycle Kicks 20 sec
5. Leg Stretch 5 sec
6. Punches 10xs
7. Butterflies 10xs
8. Bicycle Kicks 20 sec
9. Ear to Shoulder Stretch 5 sec
10. Pull-up and Sit 1 min
11. Forearm Plank 20 sec
12. Inside-Out Kicks 10xs
13. Back Stretch 5 sec
14. Sit-ups 5xs
15. Forearm Plank 10 sec
16. Chin to Floor Stretch 5 sec
17. Guided Standing 20 sec—*new exercise*
18. Chin Lift Stretch 5 sec
19. Bumbo Time 5 min

Estimated Time: 14 minutes

INCLUDED MILESTONE ACTIVITIES
On tummy, lift head 90 degrees (Tummy Time)
Hold head steady when upright (Bumbo Time/Guided Sitting)
Roll over one way (Tummy Time)
On tummy, raise chest, supported by arms (Tummy Time)

ADDITIONAL MILESTONE ACTIVITIES
Follow an object in an arc six inches above face from one
side to the other
Grasp a rattle

Month Five Workout

1. Tummy Time 5 min
2. Punches 30xs
3. Butterflies 30xs
4. Bicycle Kicks 30 sec
5. Leg Stretch 5 sec
6. Punches 15xs
7. Butterflies 15xs
8. Guided Standing 1 min
9. Bicycle Kicks 30 sec
10. Ear to Shoulder Stretch 5 sec
11. Forearm Plank 20 sec
12. Crawling Position 5 sec—*new exercise*
13. Back Stretch 5 sec
14. Pull-ups to Standing 3xs—*new exercise*
15. Plank (hold at hips) 10 sec—*new exercise*
16. Guided Standing 30 sec
17. Sit-ups 10xs
18. Chin to Floor Stretch 5 sec
19. Bumbo Time 5 min

Estimated Time: 16 minutes

INCLUDED MILESTONE ACTIVITIES
Hold head steady when upright (Guided Sitting)
On tummy, raise chest supported by arms (Tummy Time)
Roll over one way (Tummy Time)
Bear some weight on legs (Guided Standing)
Keep head level with body when pulled to sitting (Sit-ups)

ADDITIONAL MILESTONE ACTIVITIES
Grasp a rattle

Month Six Workout

1. Punches 30xs
2. Butterflies 30xs
3. Bicycle Kicks 30 sec
4. Leg Stretch 5 sec
5. Punches 20xs
6. Butterflies 20xs
7. Guided Standing 1 min
8. Sit-ups 10xs
9. Toe to Nose Touch—*new exercise*
10. Plank 15 sec (hold at hips)
11. Bicycle Kicks 30 sec
12. Crawling Position 5 sec
13. Plank 10 sec (hold at thighs)
14. Pull-ups to Standing 5xs
15. Crawling Position 5 sec
16. Back Stretch 5 sec
17. Guided Standing 1 min
18. Bumbo Time 5 min

Estimated Time: 12 minutes

INCLUDED MILESTONE ACTIVITIES
Keep head level with body when pulled to sitting (Sit-ups)
Sit without support (Guided Sitting)
Bear some weight on legs when held upright
(Guided Standing)

Month Seven Workout

1. Punches 30xs
2. Butterflies 30xs
3. Bicycle Kicks 30 sec
4. Leg Stretch 5 sec
5. Punches 25xs
6. Butterflies 25xs
7. Guided Standing 1 min
8. Sit-ups 10xs
9. Toe to Nose Touch
10. Plank 15 sec (hold at thighs)
11. Bicycle Kicks 30 sec
12. Pull-ups to Standing 5xs
13. Guided Walking 10 steps
14. Plank 10 sec (hold at knees)
15. Back Stretch 5 sec
16. Bumbo Time 5 min

Estimated Time: 11 minutes

INCLUDED MILESTONE ACTIVITIES
Sit without support (Guided Sitting)
Bear some weight on legs when held upright
(Guided Standing)

ADDITIONAL MILESTONE ACTIVITIES
Play peekaboo

Month Eight Workout

1. Punches 30xs
2. Butterflies 30xs
3. Bicycle Kicks 30 sec
4. Leg Stretch 5 sec
5. Punches 30xs
6. Butterflies 30xs
7. Guided Standing 1 min
8. Sit-ups 10xs
9. Toe to Nose Touch
10. Plank 15 sec (hold at knees)
11. Bicycle Kicks 30 sec
12. Pull-ups to Standing 5xs
13. Guided Walking 15 steps
14. Plank 15 sec (hold at knees)
15. Back Stretch 5 sec

Estimated Time: 6 minutes

INCLUDED MILESTONE ACTIVITIES
Bear some weight on legs when held upright
(Guided Standing)
Stand holding onto someone or something
(Guided Standing)

ADDITIONAL MILESTONE ACTIVITIES
Get into sitting position from tummy
(this will happen naturally from regular activity)
Play peekaboo

www.ingramcontent.com/pod-product-compliance
Lightning Source LLC
Chambersburg PA
CBHW060701280326
41933CB00012B/2259